NAVIGATING THE USE OF OMEPRAZOLE

A COMPREHENSIVE GUIDE ON THE EFFECTIVE TREATMENT OF PEPTIC ULCER

TABLE OF CONTENTS

CHAPTER 1

UNDERSTANDING PEPTIC ULCERS

1.1 What are Peptic Ulcers?

Peptic ulcers are open sores that develop on the lining of the stomach, small intestine, or esophagus. These ulcers form when the protective mucus layer that normally shields the digestive tract from stomach acid becomes weakened or damaged. As a result, the acidic digestive juices begin to erode the underlying tissues, leading to painful sores. The term "peptic" is derived from the Latin word "pepticus," which means "pertaining to digestion," highlighting the role of digestive acids in ulcer formation.

There are two main types of peptic ulcers: gastric ulcers, which occur in the stomach; and duodenal ulcers, which develop in the upper part of the small intestine known as the duodenum. Esophageal ulcers, though less common, can also occur in the esophagus. These ulcers vary in severity, with some causing minor discomfort and others leading to more serious health complications, such as bleeding or perforation.

1.2 Causes and Risk Factors

The primary causes of peptic ulcers include infection with *Helicobacter pylori* (H. pylori) bacteria and the prolonged use of nonsteroidal anti-inflammatory drugs (NSAIDs).

H. pylori Infection: This bacterium is a major contributor to peptic ulcer disease. It colonizes the mucosal lining of the stomach and duodenum, leading to inflammation and damage. H. pylori infection is common worldwide, but not everyone infected with the bacterium develops ulcers. It is believed that genetic predisposition, environmental factors, and the bacteria's ability to evade the immune system play roles in the development of ulcers.

NSAIDs: Medications such as ibuprofen, aspirin, and naproxen can impair the stomach's ability to produce mucus and bicarbonate, which are crucial for protecting the mucosal lining from acid damage. Chronic use of NSAIDs, especially in high doses, increases the risk of developing peptic ulcers. These drugs can cause irritation and inflammation, leading to ulcer formation.

Other risk factors for peptic ulcers include:

- **Excessive Alcohol Consumption**: Alcohol can irritate and erode the mucosal lining of the stomach, increasing ulcer risk. It also impairs the healing process of existing ulcers.

- **Smoking**: Nicotine and other chemicals in tobacco can increase stomach acid production and decrease the production of protective mucus, making smokers more susceptible to peptic ulcers. Smoking also impairs ulcer healing.

- **Stress**: Although stress alone does not cause peptic ulcers, it can exacerbate symptoms and interfere with healing. Stress may increase acid production and contribute to unhealthy behaviors, such as smoking or alcohol consumption, which further aggravate ulcer conditions.

- **Genetics**: A family history of peptic ulcers or related conditions may increase one's susceptibility. Certain genetic factors may influence how the body responds to H. pylori infection or NSAID use.

- **Certain Medical Conditions**: Conditions such as Zollinger-Ellison syndrome, which causes excessive acid production, can predispose individuals to peptic ulcers.

1.3 Symptoms and Diagnosis

Symptoms: The symptoms of peptic ulcers can vary depending on the ulcer's location and severity. Common symptoms include:

- **Abdominal Pain**: This is the most prevalent symptom and is often described as a burning or gnawing sensation in the upper abdomen. The pain may be relieved temporarily by eating or taking antacids but can return after a few hours.
- **Nausea and Vomiting**: Individuals with peptic ulcers may experience nausea or vomiting. In some cases, vomit may contain blood or appear coffee-ground-like due to digested blood.
- **Bloating and Belching**: A feeling of fullness or bloating after meals, along with excessive belching, is common among ulcer sufferers.
- **Loss of Appetite and Weight Loss**: Persistent abdominal discomfort and pain can lead to a decreased appetite, resulting in unintended weight loss.
- **Heartburn**: Some individuals with peptic ulcers experience symptoms similar to acid reflux or heartburn, characterized by a burning sensation in the chest.

In more severe cases, peptic ulcers can lead to complications such as:

- **Bleeding**: This can manifest as blood in the vomit or black, tarry stools. Severe bleeding may require medical intervention.
- **Perforation**: An ulcer can erode through the stomach or intestinal wall, leading to a perforation. This results in abdominal pain and requires immediate surgical treatment.
- **Obstruction**: Ulcers can cause swelling and scarring that block the passage of food through the digestive tract, leading to symptoms like persistent vomiting and bloating.

Diagnosis: To diagnose peptic ulcers, healthcare providers use a combination of medical history, physical examination, and diagnostic tests. Key diagnostic procedures include:

- **Endoscopy**: A flexible tube with a camera is inserted through the mouth to visually inspect the digestive tract. This procedure allows for direct visualization of ulcers and, if necessary, biopsy samples for further analysis.

- **Upper Gastrointestinal Series (Barium Swallow)**: This imaging test involves drinking a barium-containing liquid that coats the digestive tract, making ulcers visible on X-rays.

- **H. pylori Testing**: Tests for H. pylori infection include breath tests, stool tests, and blood tests. Breath and stool tests are non-invasive and can detect active infections, while blood tests identify antibodies against the bacteria.

- **Laboratory Tests**: Blood tests may be conducted to check for anemia or other signs of bleeding, while stool tests can identify blood in the stool.

CHAPTER 2

INTRODUCTION TO OMEPRAZOLE

2.1 What is Omeprazole?

Omeprazole is a widely used medication belonging to a class of drugs known as proton pump inhibitors (PPIs). It is primarily prescribed for the treatment of conditions related to excessive stomach acid production, such as peptic ulcers, gastroesophageal reflux disease (GERD), and Zollinger-Ellison syndrome. Omeprazole is a potent agent that helps reduce the amount of acid produced in the stomach, providing relief from symptoms and promoting the healing of acid-related damage.

The drug was first approved for use in the late 1980s and has since become one of the most commonly prescribed PPIs worldwide. It is available under various brand names, including Prilosec, and is also offered in generic form. Omeprazole has gained popularity due to its effectiveness, safety profile, and relatively low cost compared to other treatments.

2.2 How Omeprazole Works

Omeprazole's primary mechanism of action is its ability to inhibit the proton pump in the stomach. The proton pump, also known as the hydrogen-potassium ATPase, is an enzyme found in the parietal cells of the stomach lining. This enzyme is responsible for the final step in the production of gastric acid. By blocking this enzyme, omeprazole effectively reduces the amount of acid secreted into the stomach.

Here's a more detailed breakdown of how omeprazole works:

1. **Absorption and Activation**: Omeprazole is absorbed in the small intestine and then travels to the stomach. Once in the acidic environment of the parietal cells, it is converted into its active form. This activation occurs within the acidic environment of the parietal cells' canaliculi (small channels leading to the surface of the cell).

2. **Inhibition of Proton Pump**: The active form of omeprazole binds covalently to the proton pumps within the parietal cells. This binding irreversibly inhibits the enzyme's ability to secrete hydrogen ions

into the gastric lumen. Since hydrogen ions combine with chloride ions to form hydrochloric acid, the reduction in hydrogen ion secretion leads to a decrease in overall gastric acid production.

3. **Reduction in Acid Production**: By inhibiting the proton pumps, omeprazole effectively reduces the acidity of the stomach contents. This reduction in acid production helps to alleviate symptoms of acid-related disorders and promotes healing of damaged tissues.

4. **Duration of Effect**: Omeprazole provides long-lasting acid suppression due to its irreversible inhibition of the proton pumps. The drug's effects can last for up to 24 hours, and it typically takes several days of consistent use to achieve optimal therapeutic effects. New proton pumps need to be synthesized by the body to restore normal acid production, which is why it may take a few days to weeks for the full effects of the drug to be evident.

2.3 Forms and Dosage of Omeprazole

Omeprazole is available in several forms to accommodate different patient needs and treatment regimens. The most common forms include:

1. **Oral Capsules**: Omeprazole is available in delayed-release capsules, which are designed to release the medication gradually to ensure effective absorption and prolonged action. These capsules are typically taken once daily, though the dosage may vary based on the condition being treated.

2. **Oral Tablets**: The drug is also available in tablet form, often as an enteric-coated tablet that protects the medication from stomach acid, ensuring that it is released in the small intestine where it can be absorbed.

3. **Oral Suspension**: For patients who have difficulty swallowing pills or capsules, omeprazole is available as an oral suspension. This form allows the medication to be taken as a liquid, providing an alternative for those with specific needs.

4. **Intravenous (IV) Form**: In hospital settings, omeprazole may be administered intravenously for patients who require immediate or precise acid

suppression, such as those undergoing surgery or with severe acid-related conditions.

The dosage of omeprazole varies depending on the specific condition being treated and individual patient factors. Common dosages include:

- **Peptic Ulcers**: For the treatment of peptic ulcers, the typical dose is 20 mg to 40 mg once daily. The duration of treatment can range from 4 to 8 weeks, depending on the severity of the ulcer and the patient's response to the medication.

- **Gastroesophageal Reflux Disease (GERD)**: For GERD, the usual dose is 20 mg to 40 mg once daily. Treatment duration may vary but often lasts for several weeks to months, depending on symptom control and the presence of any complications.

- **H. pylori Eradication**: When used in combination with antibiotics for the eradication of *Helicobacter pylori*, the dose is typically 20 mg twice daily. The combination therapy usually lasts for 10 to 14 days.

- **Zollinger-Ellison Syndrome**: For this condition, which involves excessive acid production, the dosage can range from 60 mg to 120 mg per day, administered in divided doses. The treatment is tailored to the individual's acid production levels and response to therapy.

It is important for patients to follow their healthcare provider's instructions regarding dosage and duration of treatment. Omeprazole is usually taken before meals, and it is recommended to swallow the capsules or tablets whole without crushing or chewing, as this can affect the drug's effectiveness.

CHAPTER 3

OMEPRAZOLE IN PEPTIC ULCER TREATMENT

3.1 Mechanism of Action in Ulcer Healing

Omeprazole is an essential medication in the treatment of peptic ulcers due to its powerful mechanism of action, which primarily involves the suppression of gastric acid production. Peptic ulcers are sores that develop on the lining of the stomach, small intestine, or esophagus, primarily due to the erosion caused by excessive stomach acid. The healing of these ulcers is closely linked to the reduction of gastric acid, and omeprazole plays a crucial role in this process.

Mechanism of Action: Omeprazole is a proton pump inhibitor (PPI) that targets the proton pumps located in the parietal cells of the stomach lining. The proton pump, also known as the hydrogen-potassium ATPase, is responsible for the final step in the production of gastric acid. It actively transports hydrogen ions (protons) into the stomach lumen in exchange for potassium ions.

Omeprazole is a prodrug, meaning it requires activation to exert its effects. After oral administration, omeprazole is

16

absorbed in the small intestine and travels to the parietal cells in the stomach lining. Within the acidic environment of these cells, omeprazole is converted into its active form. The active form of omeprazole covalently binds to the proton pumps, irreversibly inhibiting their activity. This binding prevents the proton pumps from secreting hydrogen ions into the stomach, thereby reducing the production of hydrochloric acid.

By decreasing gastric acid secretion, omeprazole reduces the acidity of the stomach contents. This reduction in acid helps to:

1. **Decrease Gastric Irritation**: Lowering the acid levels in the stomach minimizes irritation and damage to the ulcerated areas, providing a more favorable environment for healing.
2. **Promote Ulcer Healing**: A less acidic environment allows the damaged mucosal lining to heal more effectively. The reduction in acid also helps alleviate symptoms such as pain and discomfort associated with ulcers.
3. **Prevent Further Damage**: By inhibiting acid secretion, omeprazole prevents further erosion of the

ulcerated areas, reducing the risk of complications such as bleeding or perforation.

The effectiveness of omeprazole in promoting ulcer healing is well-documented, making it a cornerstone of treatment for peptic ulcers.

3.2 Dosage Guidelines for Ulcers

The dosage of omeprazole for the treatment of peptic ulcers is determined based on the severity of the ulcer, the presence of any complications, and individual patient factors. Dosage guidelines are designed to maximize therapeutic benefits while minimizing potential side effects.

General Dosage Recommendations:

1. **Gastric Ulcers**: For the treatment of gastric ulcers, the standard dosage of omeprazole is 20 mg to 40 mg once daily. The specific dosage may vary depending on the severity of the ulcer and the patient's response to the medication. In some cases, a higher dose of 40 mg may be used if the ulcer is particularly severe or resistant to treatment.

2. **Duodenal Ulcers**: For duodenal ulcers, the recommended dose is typically 20 mg once daily. Similar to gastric ulcers, the dosage may be adjusted based on the ulcer's severity and the patient's clinical response.

3. **H. pylori Eradication**: When used in combination with antibiotics for the eradication of *Helicobacter pylori*, omeprazole is usually administered at a dose of 20 mg twice daily. This combination therapy is often prescribed for 10 to 14 days and aims to eliminate the bacteria that contribute to ulcer formation.

4. **NSAID-Induced Ulcers**: For ulcers induced by nonsteroidal anti-inflammatory drugs (NSAIDs), omeprazole is often prescribed at a dose of 20 mg to 40 mg once daily. The dosage may be adjusted based on the patient's specific needs and the duration of NSAID use.

Considerations: The exact dosage may vary depending on individual patient factors, such as age, weight, and the presence of other medical conditions. It is important for patients to follow their healthcare provider's instructions regarding dosage and administration to ensure optimal results.

3.3 Duration of Treatment and Monitoring

The duration of omeprazole treatment for peptic ulcers is determined by the type and severity of the ulcer, as well as the patient's response to therapy. Monitoring is essential to assess the effectiveness of treatment and to make any necessary adjustments.

Duration of Treatment:

1. **Gastric and Duodenal Ulcers**: The typical treatment duration for gastric and duodenal ulcers is 4 to 8 weeks. This timeframe is usually sufficient for the majority of ulcers to heal. In some cases, a longer duration of treatment may be required, particularly if the ulcer is not fully healed or if there are complications.

2. **H. pylori Eradication**: When used in combination with antibiotics for H. pylori eradication, omeprazole is usually administered for 10 to 14 days. This duration is designed to effectively eliminate the bacteria and allow for the healing of the ulcer.

3. **NSAID-Induced Ulcers**: For ulcers induced by NSAIDs, the treatment duration may vary depending on

the patient's ongoing use of NSAIDs. Omeprazole may be prescribed for several weeks to months, and treatment duration may be adjusted based on the resolution of symptoms and the need for continued NSAID therapy.

Monitoring:

1. **Symptom Assessment**: Patients should be regularly monitored for the resolution of ulcer symptoms, such as pain, nausea, and discomfort. Improvement in symptoms is a key indicator of the medication's effectiveness.
2. **Endoscopic Evaluation**: In some cases, healthcare providers may recommend follow-up endoscopy to assess the healing of the ulcer, particularly if there are concerns about persistent or severe ulcers.
3. **Side Effects and Adverse Reactions**: Monitoring for potential side effects is important to ensure patient safety. Common side effects of omeprazole include headache, nausea, and diarrhea. Serious adverse reactions, although rare, should be promptly reported to a healthcare provider.
4. **Long-Term Use**: For patients requiring long-term omeprazole therapy, such as those with chronic

conditions or recurrent ulcers, regular monitoring is essential to assess the need for ongoing treatment and to evaluate for potential complications, such as vitamin deficiencies or bone health issues.

CHAPTER 4

POTENTIAL SIDE EFFECTS AND INTERACTIONS

4.1 Common Side Effects

Omeprazole, like all medications, can cause side effects. While many people tolerate it well, it is important to be aware of common side effects and discuss any concerns with a healthcare provider. Common side effects of omeprazole include:

1. **Headache**: One of the most frequently reported side effects, headaches can range from mild to moderate in intensity. This is generally a temporary issue that may resolve as the body adjusts to the medication.

2. **Nausea and Vomiting**: Omeprazole can cause gastrointestinal discomfort, including nausea and vomiting. These symptoms are often mild and may improve over time. If they persist or become severe, it's important to consult a healthcare provider.

3. **Diarrhea**: Another common side effect, diarrhea can occur as the medication affects the stomach's acid balance. It is usually mild but can be bothersome. Staying hydrated and eating a balanced diet may help manage this symptom.

4. **Constipation**: Some individuals may experience constipation while taking omeprazole. Increasing fiber intake and drinking plenty of fluids can help alleviate this issue.

5. **Abdominal Pain**: Mild abdominal pain or discomfort is also reported by some users. This side effect is generally not severe and tends to resolve as the body adapts to the medication.

6. **Flatulence**: Gas and bloating can occur as a side effect of omeprazole. This is usually not a serious issue but can be uncomfortable for some individuals.
7. **Dizziness**: Dizziness or lightheadedness can occasionally occur. Patients experiencing these symptoms should be cautious when performing tasks that require alertness, such as driving.
8. **Fatigue**: Some individuals may feel unusually tired or fatigued while on omeprazole. This side effect is usually mild and should improve over time.

Most of these side effects are generally mild and may diminish as the treatment continues. However, if any side effects persist or worsen, it is advisable to consult a healthcare provider.

4.2 Serious Adverse Reactions

While serious adverse reactions to omeprazole are rare, they can occur and require immediate medical attention. Serious side effects include:

1. **Allergic Reactions**: Although uncommon, some individuals may experience severe allergic reactions to

omeprazole. Symptoms can include rash, itching, swelling (especially of the face, tongue, or throat), severe dizziness, and trouble breathing. These reactions require prompt medical intervention.

2. **Clostridium difficile Infection**: Prolonged use of omeprazole can increase the risk of Clostridium difficile infection in the colon. This bacterial infection can cause severe diarrhea, abdominal pain, and fever. It requires treatment with antibiotics and, in severe cases, hospitalization.

3. **Kidney Problems**: Rarely, omeprazole can lead to kidney issues, including acute interstitial nephritis, which is an inflammation of the kidney's interstitial tissue. Symptoms may include swelling, decreased urine output, and blood in the urine. Monitoring kidney function during long-term therapy may be necessary.

4. **Bone Fractures**: Long-term use of omeprazole has been associated with an increased risk of bone fractures, particularly in the hip, wrist, and spine. This is thought to be related to decreased calcium absorption. Patients on prolonged therapy should be monitored for bone health and may need calcium and vitamin D supplements.

5. **Low Magnesium Levels**: Omeprazole can cause hypomagnesemia (low magnesium levels) if used for extended periods. Symptoms of low magnesium include muscle spams, irregular heartbeat, and seizures. Regular monitoring of magnesium levels may be necessary during long-term therapy.

6. **Lupus Erythematosus**: Although rare, omeprazole has been linked to drug-induced lupus erythematosus, a condition characterized by symptoms such as rash, joint pain, and fever. Discontinuation of the medication usually leads to resolution of symptoms.

7. **Severe Liver Issues**: In very rare cases, omeprazole may lead to severe liver damage, evidenced by jaundice (yellowing of the skin or eyes), dark urine, and severe fatigue. Liver function tests should be monitored if symptoms suggest liver impairment.

Patients experiencing any of these serious adverse reactions should seek immediate medical attention to address the issues and discuss alternative treatment options if necessary.

4.3 Drug Interactions and Precautions

Omeprazole can interact with various medications, potentially affecting their efficacy or increasing the risk of side effects. Understanding these interactions is crucial for safe and effective use of the medication. Key drug interactions and precautions include:

1. **Clopidogrel**: Omeprazole can interfere with the activation of clopidogrel, an antiplatelet medication used to prevent blood clots. This interaction can reduce the effectiveness of clopidogrel, increasing the risk of cardiovascular events. Alternatives or dose adjustments may be necessary.

2. **Warfarin**: Omeprazole can affect the metabolism of warfarin, an anticoagulant, potentially altering its effectiveness and increasing the risk of bleeding. Regular monitoring of INR (International Normalized Ratio) levels is recommended for patients taking both medications.

3. **Diazepam**: Omeprazole may increase the levels of diazepam, a medication used for anxiety and seizures, by inhibiting its metabolism. This can enhance the effects and side effects of diazepam. Dose adjustments and careful monitoring are advisable.

4. **Methotrexate**: Omeprazole can increase the levels of methotrexate, a drug used for cancer and autoimmune diseases, leading to potential toxicity. Caution is needed, and dose adjustments may be required for patients on high-dose methotrexate therapy.

5. **Atazanavir**: Omeprazole can reduce the absorption of atazanavir, an antiretroviral medication used for HIV treatment. This interaction can decrease the effectiveness of atazanavir. Alternative treatments or dosage adjustments may be necessary.

6. **Digoxin**: Omeprazole can increase digoxin levels, a medication used for heart conditions, potentially leading to toxicity. Monitoring of digoxin levels is recommended to avoid adverse effects.

7. **Vitamin and Mineral Absorption**: Long-term use of omeprazole may affect the absorption of certain vitamins and minerals, including vitamin B12, calcium, and magnesium. Patients on long-term therapy should be monitored for deficiencies and may require supplementation.

Precautions:

- **Pregnancy and Breastfeeding**: Omeprazole is classified as a Category C drug during pregnancy, meaning that its use should be considered only if the potential benefits outweigh the risks. It is also excreted in breast milk, so caution is advised for breastfeeding mothers. Alternative treatments should be discussed with a healthcare provider.

- **Pre-existing Conditions**: Patients with pre-existing liver conditions or kidney issues should use omeprazole with caution. Dose adjustments and regular monitoring may be required.
- **Long-term Use**: For patients requiring long-term omeprazole therapy, regular monitoring of bone health, magnesium levels, and kidney function is essential to minimize the risk of complications.

CHAPTER 5

COMBINING OMEPRAZOLE WITH OTHER
THERAPIES

5.1 Antibiotic Therapy for H. pylori Eradication

Helicobacter pylori (*H. pylori*) is a gram-negative bacterium that plays a central role in the development of peptic ulcers and chronic gastritis. To effectively manage ulcers, especially those associated with *H. pylori*, combination therapy is often employed, incorporating omeprazole along with antibiotics. This approach is designed to eradicate the infection and promote ulcer healing.

Standard Triple Therapy: The most common regimen for *H. pylori* eradication is the triple therapy, which includes:

1. **Omeprazole**: Typically administered at a dose of 20 mg to 40 mg twice daily. Omeprazole helps reduce gastric acid secretion, creating a less acidic environment that enhances the effectiveness of antibiotics.

2. **Antibiotics**: The standard antibiotics used are amoxicillin and clarithromycin. Amoxicillin is usually

given at a dose of 1 g twice daily, while clarithromycin is administered at a dose of 500 mg twice daily. These antibiotics work synergistically to kill *H. pylori* and prevent resistance.

3. **Additional Antibiotic**: In some cases, a third antibiotic, such as metronidazole (500 mg twice daily) or tetracycline (500 mg four times daily), is added to the regimen, especially in areas with high rates of antibiotic resistance.

Duration of Therapy: The typical duration of triple therapy is 10 to 14 days. Adherence to the full course is crucial to ensure the eradication of *H. pylori* and prevent recurrence. The effectiveness of the treatment is monitored through follow-up testing, such as a urea breath test, stool antigen test, or endoscopy with biopsy.

Quadruple Therapy: In cases of resistance to clarithromycin or failure of triple therapy, quadruple therapy may be used. This regimen includes:

1. **Omeprazole**: 20 mg to 40 mg twice daily.
2. **Bismuth Subsalicylate**: 525 mg four times daily. Bismuth helps protect the stomach lining and has mild antimicrobial properties.

3. **Metronidazole**: 250 mg to 500 mg three to four times daily.

4. **Tetracycline**: 500 mg four times daily.

Effectiveness: Combination therapy with omeprazole and antibiotics is highly effective in eradicating *H. pylori* and healing associated ulcers. Successful eradication of the bacterium is linked to a significant reduction in ulcer recurrence and improvement in symptoms.

5.2 Lifestyle and Dietary Modifications

In addition to pharmacological treatments, lifestyle and dietary modifications play a vital role in the management of peptic ulcers. These changes can enhance the effectiveness of omeprazole and reduce ulcer symptoms.

Dietary Adjustments:

1. **Avoid Irritants**: Foods and beverages that can irritate the stomach lining or increase acid production should be minimized. These include spicy foods, caffeine, alcohol, and carbonated drinks. Avoiding these can help reduce symptoms and promote healing.

2. **Eat Smaller, More Frequent Meals**: Eating smaller meals more frequently can help prevent excessive acid production and reduce the burden on the stomach. This approach can help manage symptoms and prevent exacerbations.

3. **Incorporate Alkaline Foods**: Foods that help neutralize stomach acid, such as bananas, oatmeal, and non-citrus fruits, can be beneficial. These foods can provide relief from acidity and promote a more balanced gastric environment.

4. **Increase Fiber Intake**: A diet high in fiber, particularly from fruits, vegetables, and whole grains, can support digestive health and reduce ulcer symptoms. Fiber aids in digestion and can help reduce acid production.

Lifestyle Changes:

1. **Quit Smoking**: Smoking can impair the healing of peptic ulcers and increase acid production. Quitting smoking is a crucial step in managing ulcers and improving overall health.

2. **Reduce Alcohol Consumption**: Alcohol can irritate the stomach lining and exacerbate ulcer symptoms.

Limiting or avoiding alcohol can aid in ulcer healing and reduce discomfort.

3. **Manage Stress**: Stress does not cause ulcers directly but can aggravate symptoms and hinder healing. Stress management techniques, such as mindfulness, relaxation exercises, and regular physical activity, can be beneficial.

4. **Exercise Regularly**: Regular, moderate exercise can help manage stress and support overall digestive health. Activities like walking, swimming, or cycling can promote well-being and potentially reduce ulcer symptoms.

5. **Avoid NSAIDs**: Nonsteroidal anti-inflammatory drugs (NSAIDs) can exacerbate ulcer symptoms and interfere with healing. If pain management is necessary, alternative medications or therapies should be discussed with a healthcare provider.

5.3 Alternative and Complementary Treatments

In addition to conventional therapies, some individuals explore alternative and complementary treatments to manage peptic ulcers. These approaches can sometimes provide additional benefits or support alongside standard treatment with omeprazole.

Herbal Remedies:

1. **Licorice Root**: Deglycyrrhizinated licorice (DGL) is a form of licorice root that has been used to promote ulcer healing. It is thought to have mucosal-protective properties and may help soothe the stomach lining. DGL is typically available as a chewable tablet.

2. **Slippery Elm**: Slippery elm contains mucilage, which forms a soothing gel-like substance when mixed with water. This mucilage can coat and protect the stomach lining, potentially providing relief from ulcer symptoms.

3. **Marshmallow Root**: Similar to slippery elm, marshmallow root contains mucilage that can help soothe and protect the gastrointestinal tract. It is available in various forms, including teas and capsules.

4. **Turmeric**: Curcumin, the active compound in turmeric, has anti-inflammatory and antioxidant properties. Some studies suggest that turmeric may help reduce inflammation and promote healing in the digestive tract.

Probiotics:

Probiotics are beneficial bacteria that support gut health. They may help restore balance to the gut microbiota, which can be disrupted by antibiotic therapy. Probiotics, such as Lactobacillus and Bifidobacterium strains, can be found in yogurt and dietary supplements. They may help alleviate gastrointestinal symptoms and support overall digestive health.

Acupuncture:

Acupuncture, a traditional Chinese medicine practice, involves inserting fine needles into specific points on the body to promote healing and balance. Some studies suggest that acupuncture may help reduce ulcer symptoms, improve digestion, and manage stress.

Mind-Body Therapies:

Techniques such as mindfulness meditation, yoga, and guided imagery can help manage stress and improve overall well-being. While not a direct treatment for ulcers, these therapies can complement conventional treatment by reducing stress and supporting mental health.

Nutritional Supplements:

1. **Vitamin C**: Vitamin C is known for its role in collagen synthesis and wound healing. Supplementing with vitamin C may support the healing process of ulcers.
2. **Zinc**: Zinc is essential for cell growth and repair. Some studies suggest that zinc supplementation may help promote ulcer healing.
3. **Omega-3 Fatty Acids**: Found in fish oil, omega-3 fatty acids have anti-inflammatory properties and may support gastrointestinal health.

Caution: While alternative and complementary treatments can provide additional support, they should not replace conventional therapies such as omeprazole or antibiotics. It is essential to discuss any alternative treatments with a healthcare provider to ensure they are safe and appropriate for individual health needs.

CHAPTER 6

CONCLUSION AND FUTURE PERSPECTIVES

6.1 Summary of Key Points

The effective treatment of peptic ulcers involves a multifaceted approach that includes the use of medications, lifestyle modifications, and sometimes alternative therapies. Omeprazole, a widely used proton pump inhibitor (PPI), plays a central role in managing peptic ulcers by reducing gastric acid production and promoting ulcer healing. Here's a summary of the key points covered in this guide:

1. **Understanding Peptic Ulcers**: Peptic ulcers are sores that develop on the lining of the stomach, small intestine, or esophagus. They are often caused by an infection with *Helicobacter pylori* or by the use of nonsteroidal anti-inflammatory drugs (NSAIDs). Symptoms include abdominal pain, bloating, nausea, and in severe cases, bleeding.

2. **Introduction to Omeprazole**: Omeprazole is a PPI that works by irreversibly inhibiting the proton pumps in the stomach lining, thus reducing the secretion of gastric acid. It is available in various forms and dosages,

typically administered once or twice daily, depending on the condition being treated.

3. **Omeprazole in Peptic Ulcer Treatment**: Omeprazole's mechanism of action is crucial for ulcer healing as it creates a less acidic environment, promoting mucosal repair. Dosage guidelines generally range from 20 mg to 40 mg daily, and treatment duration varies based on the ulcer's severity and response. Regular monitoring is necessary to ensure effective treatment and to manage any potential side effects.

4. **Potential Side Effects and Interactions**: While omeprazole is effective, it can cause common side effects such as headache, nausea, and diarrhea. Serious adverse reactions, though rare, include allergic reactions and kidney problems. Drug interactions with medications like clopidogrel and warfarin are also important considerations. Patients should be aware of these potential issues and discuss any concerns with their healthcare provider.

5. **Combining Omeprazole with Other Therapies**: Combining omeprazole with antibiotic therapy is often necessary to eradicate *H. pylori*. Lifestyle and dietary modifications, such as avoiding irritants and managing

stress, can further support ulcer healing. Alternative treatments, including herbal remedies and probiotics, may complement conventional therapies but should be used under professional guidance.

6.2 Ongoing Research and Developments

Research in the field of gastroenterology is continually advancing, aiming to improve the management of peptic ulcers and the efficacy of treatments like omeprazole. Some of the key areas of ongoing research and developments include:

1. **Enhanced PPIs**: New PPIs are being developed to offer more targeted action or reduced side effects compared to existing options. These include medications with different pharmacokinetic profiles that might offer longer-lasting or more effective acid suppression.
2. **Resistance to *H. pylori***: Research is focusing on understanding and overcoming resistance to *H. pylori* treatment. This includes developing new antibiotics and

alternative therapeutic strategies to address resistant strains of the bacterium.

3. **Biologic Therapies**: Innovative treatments, such as biologic therapies, are being explored to target the inflammatory processes involved in ulcer formation. These therapies may provide new options for patients who do not respond well to conventional treatments.

4. **Personalized Medicine**: Advances in genomics and personalized medicine are allowing for more tailored treatment approaches. Research is investigating how genetic factors influence ulcer development and treatment responses, which may lead to personalized treatment regimens in the future.

5. **Long-Term Effects of PPIs**: There is ongoing research into the long-term effects of prolonged PPI use, including potential impacts on bone health, kidney function, and gut microbiota. This research aims to better understand the risks and benefits of long-term PPI therapy and to develop strategies to mitigate any adverse effects.

6. **Alternative Therapies**: Studies are being conducted to evaluate the effectiveness and safety of various alternative and complementary therapies, including new herbal remedies, dietary supplements, and lifestyle

interventions. This research aims to provide evidence-based recommendations for integrating these approaches into conventional treatment plans.

6.3 Final Thoughts and Recommendations

In conclusion, managing peptic ulcers effectively requires a comprehensive approach that includes pharmacological treatment, lifestyle adjustments, and, when appropriate, complementary therapies. Omeprazole remains a cornerstone of ulcer treatment due to its potent acid-suppressing properties. However, its use must be carefully managed to balance benefits with potential risks and side effects.

Final Thoughts:

- **Integrated Care**: An integrated approach that combines omeprazole with antibiotic therapy for *H. pylori* eradication, lifestyle and dietary changes, and potentially complementary treatments offers the best chance for successful ulcer management. This holistic approach addresses not only the symptoms but also the underlying causes of ulcers.

- **Patient-Centered Care**: Treatment plans should be individualized based on each patient's specific needs, preferences, and health conditions. Regular follow-up and communication between patients and healthcare providers are essential to monitor progress, manage side effects, and adjust treatment as needed.

- **Education and Awareness**: Educating patients about their condition, treatment options, and the importance of adherence to therapy can improve outcomes. Patients should be informed about potential side effects, drug interactions, and the significance of lifestyle modifications.

Recommendations:

1. **Adherence to Treatment**: Patients should follow their prescribed treatment regimen diligently and complete the full course of therapy, especially when treating *H. pylori* infections. Non-adherence can lead to treatment failure and recurrence of ulcers.

2. **Regular Monitoring**: Regular monitoring of treatment effectiveness and potential side effects is crucial, particularly for patients on long-term omeprazole therapy. This includes monitoring for any adverse effects and assessing the need for ongoing treatment.

3. **Lifestyle Modifications**: Patients should be encouraged to make lifestyle and dietary changes that support ulcer healing and prevent recurrence. This includes avoiding irritants, managing stress, and adopting a balanced diet.

4. **Discuss Alternative Therapies**: Patients interested in alternative or complementary treatments should discuss these options with their healthcare provider to ensure they are safe and do not interfere with conventional therapies.

5. **Stay Informed**: Both patients and healthcare providers should stay informed about new research and developments in the field of ulcer treatment. This knowledge can lead to more effective and personalized treatment strategies.

Omeprazole is an effective treatment for peptic ulcers, a comprehensive and patient-centered approach is essential for optimal management. Ongoing research and developments in the field offer promising advancements that may enhance treatment options and improve patient outcomes in the future.